Sirtfood Diet Recipes for Man

The Full Recipe Book For Man To Increase Metabolic Process, Drop Weight As Well As Obtain Lean Swiftly

by Micah Gordon

Sommario

Introduction

The Sirtfood Diet regimen is based upon foods that promote sirtuins, the supposed slimness genetics. These genetics are specifically reliable at melting fat as well as fixing cells while boosting wellness.

Unlike various other diet regimens that often tend to get rid of food, the Sirt diet regimen contains choosing the best foods as well as enables you to shed 3 kg weekly without unneeded sacrifices.

This diet plan contains 2 stages:

Stage 1) Throughout the very first one that lasts 7 days, in the very early 3 days, you take in an optimum of 10000 calories daily; from the 4th to the 7th day, you take in 1500 calories.

Stage 2) Lasts 2 week as well as is the upkeep.

In this publication, you will certainly discover dishes to attempt; I suggest having a diet regimen strategy prepared by a physician or a seasoned nutritional expert. I likewise advise a light exercise.

Chapter 1 Breakfast Recipes

Blueberry Frozen Yogurt

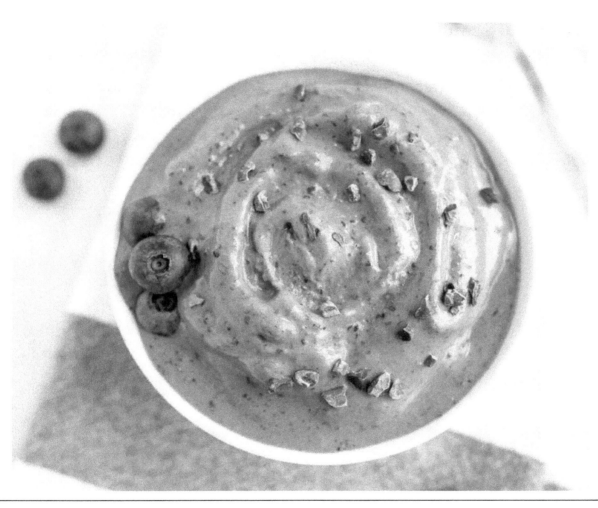

Preparation time: 1 hour 10 minutes
Cooking time: 0 minutes
Servings: 4

Ingredients: 1 teaspoon honey

450g plain yogurt 175g blueberries Juice of 1 orange

Directions: Place the blueberries and orange juice into a food processor or blender and blitz until smooth. Press the mixture through a sieve into a large bowl to remove seeds. Stir in the honey and yogurt. Transfer the mixture to an ice-cream maker and follow the manufacturer's instructions. Alternatively pour the mixture into a container and place in the fridge for 1 hour. Use a fork to whisk it and break up ice crystals and freeze for 2 hours.

Nutrition: Calories: 66 Net carbs: 8.3g Protein: 8.2g

Vegetable & Nut Loaf

Preparation time: 15 minutes
Cooking time: 1 hour 45 minutes
Servings: 4

Ingredients:

175g mushrooms, finely chopped

100g haricot beans

100g walnuts, finely chopped

100g peanuts, finely chopped

1 carrot, finely chopped

3 sticks celery, finely chopped

1 bird's-eye chili, finely chopped

1 red onion, finely chopped

1 egg, beaten

2 cloves garlic, chopped

2 teaspoons olive oil

2 teaspoons turmeric powder

2teaspoonss soy sauce

4g fresh parsley, chopped

100mls water

60mls red wine

Directions:

Heat the oil in a pan and add the garlic, chili, carrot, celery, onion, mushrooms and turmeric. Cook for 5 minutes. Place the haricot beans in a bowl and stir in the nuts, vegetables, soy sauce, egg, parsley, red wine and water. Grease and line a large loaf tin with greaseproof paper. Spoon the mixture into the loaf tin, cover with foil and bake in the oven at 190C/375F for 60-90 minutes. Let it stand for 10 minutes then turn onto a serving plate.

Nutrition:

Calories: 280

Net carbs: 29.7g

Fat: 16.3g

Fiber: 1.2g

Protein: 4.6g

Dates & Parma Ham

Preparation time: 15 minutes
Cooking time: 0 minutes
Servings: 4

Ingredients:

12 medjool dates

2 slices Parma ham, cut into strips

Directions:

Wrap each date with a strip of Parma ham. Can be served hot or cold.

Nutrition:

Calories: 202

Net carbs: 17.9g

Protein: 0.4G

Braised Celery

Preparation time: 15 minutes
Cooking time: 15 minutes
Servings: 4

Ingredients:

250g celery, chopped

100mls warm vegetable stock (broth)

1 red onion, chopped

1 clove of garlic, crushed

1 fresh parsley, chopped

25g butter

Sea salt and freshly ground black pepper

Directions:

Place the celery, onion, stock (broth) and garlic into a saucepan and bring it to the boil, reduce the heat and simmer for 10 minutes. Stir in the parsley and butter and season with salt and pepper. Serve as an accompaniment to roast meat dishes.

Nutrition:

Calories: 367 Net carbs: 5.9g Fat: 0.2g Fiber: 2.4g

Protein: 1.2g

Cheesy Buckwheat Cakes

Preparation time: 15 minutes
Cooking time: 10 minutes
Servings: 2

Ingredients:

100g buckwheat, cooked and cooled

1 large egg 25g cheddar cheese, grated (shredded)

25g (1oz) whole meal breadcrumbs   2 shallots, chopped

2 s fresh parsley, chopped   1 olive oil

Directions:

Crack the egg into a bowl, whisk it then set aside. In a separate bowl combine all the buckwheat, cheese, shallots and parsley and mix well. Pour in the beaten egg to the buckwheat mixture and stir well. Shape the mixture into patties. Scatter the breadcrumbs on a plate and roll the patties in them. Heat the olive oil in a large frying pan and gently place the cakes in the oil. Cook for 3-4 minutes on either side until slightly golden.

Nutrition:

Calories: 358 Net carbs: 121.5g Fat: 5,7g Fiber: 17g Protein: 22.5g

Red Chicory & Stilton Cheese Boats

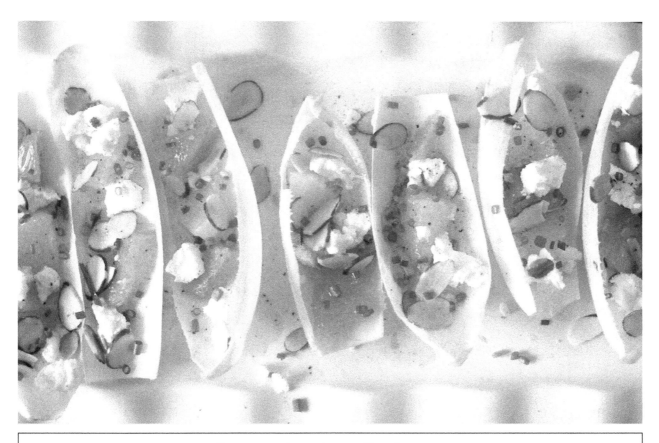

Preparation time: 5 minutes
Cooking time: 4 minutes
Servings: 4

Ingredients:

200g stilton cheese, crumbled

200g red chicory leaves (or if unavailable, use yellow)

2 fresh parsley, chopped

1 olive oil

Directions:

Place the red chicory leaves onto a baking sheet. Drizzle them with olive oil then sprinkle the cheese inside the leaves. Place them under a hot grill (broiler) for around 4 minutes until the cheese has melted. Sprinkle with chopped parsley and serve straight away.

Nutrition:

Calories: 250

Net carbs: 0.9g

Protein: 0.2g

Strawberry, Rocket (Arugula) & Feta Salad

Preparation time: 10 minutes
Cooking time: 0 minutes
Servings: 2

Ingredients:

75g fresh rocket (arugula) leaves

75g feta cheese, crumbled

100g strawberries, halved

8 walnut halves

2 spoons flaxseeds

Directions:

Combine all the ingredients in a bowl then scatter them onto two plates. For an extra Sirt food boost you can drizzle over some olive oil.

Nutrition:

Calories: 268

Net carbs: 1.1g

Fat: 6

Protein: 4g

Diced Seitan and Lentils

Preparation time: 5 minutes
Cooking time: 5 minutes
Servings: 2

Ingredients:

4 slices seitan 1 box lentils Half onion 1spoon soy cream

Salt and pepper 1 tablespoon extra-virgin olive oil

A handful of fresh parsley Turmeric (optional)

Directions: Cut the seitan into cubes. Chop the onion and brown it in oil. When it is well colored - but not burnt - add the seitan cubes and, after a few minutes, the lentils drained and well washed. Add salt and pepper and sauté with a little hot water. Finish with the cream, turmeric and chopped parsley, cook a few more minutes and then serve with a nice fresh salad and toasted whole meal bread.

Nutrition: Calories: 323 Net carbs: 36.7g Fat: 13.2g Fiber: 14.5g Protein: 16.4g

Power Cereals

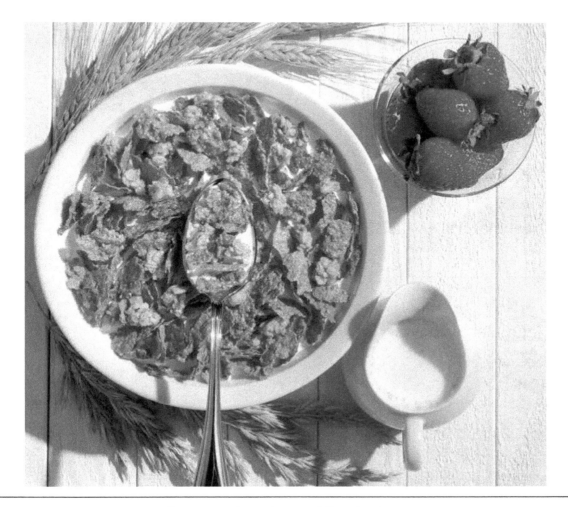

Preparation time: 10 minutes
Cooking time: 0 minutes
Servings: 1

Ingredients:

20g buckwheat flakes

10g puffed buckwheat

15g coconut flakes

40g Medjool dates, seeded and chopped

10g cocoa nibs

100g strawberries

100g Greek natural yoghurt

Directions:

Mix all ingredients together.

Nutrition:

Calories: 124g Net carbs: 27.4g Fat: 1.1g

Fiber: 1.7g Protein: 2.3g

Berry Yoghurt

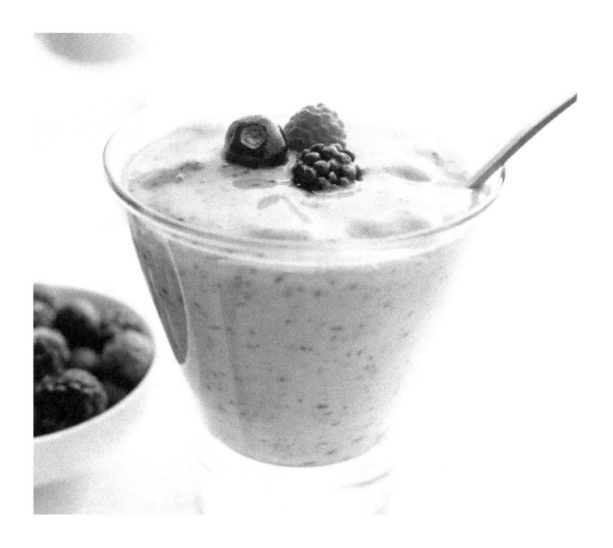

Preparation time: 10 minutes
Cooking time: 0 minutes
Servings: 1

Ingredients:

125g mixed berries 150g Greek yoghurt   25g walnuts, chopped

10g dark chocolate (85%)

Directions:

Simply mix all ingredients together.

Nutrition:

Calories: 115 Net carbs: 22.5g Fat: 1.2g Fiber: 1.1g Protein: 3g

Diced Tofu and Lentils

Preparation time: 15 minutes
Cooking time: 1 hour 20 minutes
Servings: 2

Ingredients:

200g tofu cake Soy sauce (shoyu) Extra virgin olive oil An onion

A sprig of rosemary 2 tablespoons chopped chili pepper 50g red lentils

Vegetable stock Breadcrumbs

Directions:

Marinate the diced tofu for half an hour in the soy sauce, adding a little water to cover it. In the meantime, boil the red lentils, previously washed, in the vegetable stock for about 20 minutes, until they are soft enough and the stock has dried a bit. Then sauté 2 s of chili pepper, the diced onion and rosemary in olive oil until the onion is golden brown and the sauté takes on the smell of spices. Add the tofu with some of the marinating shoyu and after a few minutes also the lentils with very little broth. Let everything shrink with the lid and over low heat and to thicken add 2 s of breadcrumbs.

Nutrition:

Calories: 141 Net carbs: 6.5g Fat: 10.8g Fiber: 0.8g Protein: 5.1g

Beans on the Bird

Preparation time: 10 minutes

Cooking time: 25 minutes

Servings: 1

Ingredients:

2 cloves of garlic, minced

2 sage leaves

2 teaspoons extra virgin olive oil

Boiled cannellini beans

Fresh well ripe tomatoes

Salt and pepper

Directions:

Brown for 2-3 minutes in a pan with oil, garlic and sage. Then add the tomatoes, cut into segments, and let them brown for a couple of minutes. Add the beans, salt and pepper to taste, stir. Cook in a covered pot for 20 minutes, checking and turning occasionally. Serve hot.

Nutrition:

Calories: 153 Net carbs: 6.6g Fiber: 2.8g Protein: 3.4g

White Beans with Lemon

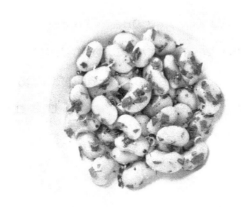

Preparation time: 5 minutes
Cooking time: 10 minutes
Servings: 1

Ingredients:

A jar of white beans from Spain

Breadcrumbs

Lemons (at least 4 but even more according to taste!)

A teaspoon of extra virgin olive oil

A big onion

Directions:

Cut the onion into fillets, put them in a pan with a little water and oil and cook. After a few minutes add the beans (rinse well under the tap). Stir and let it cook for a few minutes. Add salt, oil and breadcrumbs and mix. After a while, pour the lemon juice. Wait a little longer... and the dish is ready. Add more lemon at the end of cooking and eat!

Nutrition:

Calories: 314 Net carbs: 51.6g Fat: 2.5g Fiber: 9.9g Protein: 14.1g

Sponge Beans with Onion

Preparation time: 10 minutes
Cooking time: 3 hours
Servings: 2

Ingredients:

250 g boiled Spanish beans

1 red onion

1 parsley

Salt

2 teaspoons oil

1 teaspoon apple vinegar

1 teaspoon dried oregano or 5 fresh oregano leaves

Directions:

Cut the onion into thin slices and cook it for a minute with water in the microwave at full power. Combine all the ingredients in a bowl and leave to rest a couple of hours before serving, stirring a couple of times so that the beans take on the flavor of the seasoning.

Nutrition:

Calories: 832 Net carbs: 23.1g Fat: 11.1g Fiber: 13.9g Protein: 38.1g

Chickling Falafel

Preparation time: 24 hours
Cooking time: 30 minutes
Servings: 2

Ingredients:

Half onion 200 grams Chickling peas already soaked

80g of chickpea flour A teaspoon of cumin seed

A clove of garlic

Paprika

Directions:

Blend the chickling peas (previously soaked for 24 hours) together with the chopped onion, cumin, paprika, and garlic and chickpea flour. Blend until a fairly homogeneous mixture is obtained. Compact in a bowl and leave to rest in the fridge for about an hour. Take the dough and form some meatballs that will be baked in the oven at 180 degrees until golden brown. Notes Cumin can be reduced or eliminated completely.

Nutrition:

Calories: 57 Net carbs: 5.4g Fat: 3g Protein: 2.2g

Chickpeas and Potato Omelette

Preparation time: 10 minutes
Cooking time: 25 minutes
Servings: 2

Ingredients:

4 teaspoons full of chickpea flour

Olive oil

Small potatoes

Directions:

This dish is very similar to the traditional 'omelette', but it is better and less heavy. It can be made with any vegetable, as well as potatoes (zucchini, spinach, onion, carrots, etc.).

Put the chickpea flour in a soup plate, add 2 pinches of salt, and a little at a time water, stirring with a fork, until the dough is not too thick.

Cut the potatoes into very thin slices, with the special blade of the grater or potato peeler, and pour them into the batter, stirring well.

Put a little olive oil in a non-stick frying pan and heat over high heat.

When the oil is hot, pour the mixture, quickly distribute it evenly and put the lid on, leaving the heat high.

Both the lid and the lively fire are important to get an omelette cooked to perfection!

After about a minute, you have to turn the omelette: you can do it, if you are not able to turn it all over, by cutting it with a wooden shovel, in four slices, and turning one slice at a time.

Put the lid back on for one more minute, leaving the fire lower.

Then remove the lid, turn the omelette again and cook over high heat for one minute without lid, then turn again and cook for another minute, or until the omelette is golden on both sides.

Nutrition:

Calories: 198

Net carbs:

Fat: 4.4g

Fiber: 8.4g

Protein: 5.3g

Chapter 2 Lunch Recipes

Tuna and Tomatoes

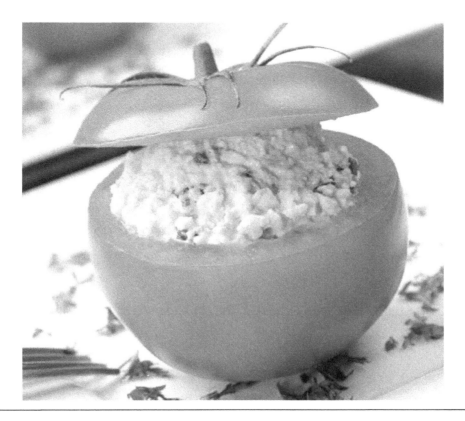

Preparation time: 5 minutes
Cooking time: 20 minutes
Servings: 4

Ingredients:

1 yellow onion, chopped

1 tablespoon olive oil

1 pound tuna fillets, boneless, skinless and cubed

1 cup tomatoes, chopped

1 red pepper, chopped

1 teaspoon sweet paprika

1 tablespoon coriander, chopped

Directions:

Heat up a pan with the oil over medium heat, add the onions and the pepper and cook for 5 minutes.

Add the fish and the other ingredients, cook everything for 15 minutes, divide between plates and serve.

Nutrition:

Calories: 215

Fat: 4g

Fiber: 7g

Carbs: 14g

Protein: 7g

Tuna and Kale

Preparation time: 5 minutes
Cooking time: 20 minutes
Servings: 4

Ingredients:

1 pound tuna fillets, boneless, skinless and cubed

A pinch of salt and black pepper

2 tablespoons olive oil

1 cup kale, torn

½ cup cherry tomatoes, cubed

1 yellow onion, chopped

Directions:

Heat up a pan with the oil over medium heat, add the onion and sauté for 5 minutes.

Add the tuna and the other ingredients, toss, cook everything for 15 minutes more, divide between plates and serve.

Nutrition:

Calories 251 Fat: 4g

Fiber: 7g Carbs: 14g Protein: 7g

Lemongrass and Ginger Mackerel

Preparation time: 10 minutes
Cooking time: 25 minutes
Servings: 4

Ingredients:

4 mackerel fillets, skinless and boneless

2 tablespoons olive oil

1 tablespoon ginger, grated

2 lemongrass sticks, chopped

2 red chilies, chopped

Juice of 1 lime

A handful parsley, chopped

Directions:

In a roasting pan, combine the mackerel with the oil, ginger and the other ingredients, toss and bake at 390 degrees F for 25 minutes.

Divide everything between plates and serve.

Nutrition:

Calories: 251

Fat: 3g

Fiber: 4g

Carbs: 14g

Protein: 8g

Scallops with Almonds and Mushrooms

Preparation time: 5 minutes
Cooking time: 10 minutes
Servings: 4

Ingredients:

1 pound scallops

2 tablespoons olive oil

4 scallions, chopped

A pinch of salt and black pepper

½ cup mushrooms, sliced

2 tablespoon almonds, chopped

1 cup coconut cream

Directions:

Heat up a pan with the oil over medium heat, add the scallions and the mushrooms and sauté for 2 minutes.

Add the scallops and the other ingredients, toss, cook over medium heat for 8 minutes more, divide into bowls and serve.

Nutrition:

Calories: 322

Fat: 23.7g

Fiber: 2.2g

Carbs: 8.1g

Protein: 21.6g

Scallops and Sweet Potatoes

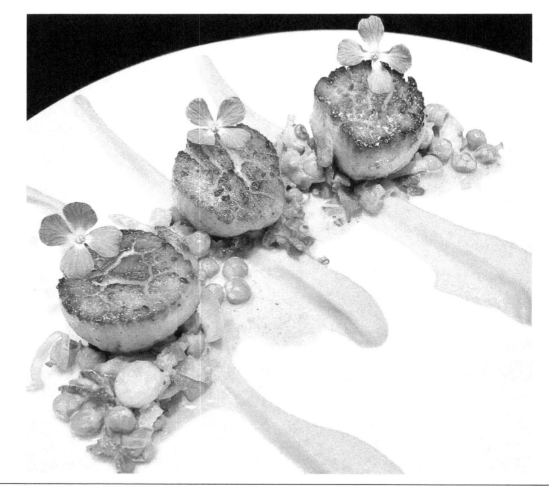

Preparation time: 5 minutes
Cooking time: 22 minutes
Servings: 4

Ingredients:

1 pound scallops

½ teaspoon rosemary, dried

½ teaspoon oregano, dried

2 tablespoons avocado oil

1 yellow onion, chopped

2 sweet potatoes, peeled and cubed

½ cup chicken stock

1 tablespoon cilantro, chopped

A pinch of salt and black pepper

Directions:

Heat up a pan with the oil over medium heat, add the onion and sauté for 2 minutes.

Add the sweet potatoes and the stock, toss and cook for 10 minutes more.

Add the scallops and the remaining ingredients, toss, cook for another 10 minutes, divide everything into bowls and serve.

Nutrition:

Calories: 211

Fat: 2g Fiber: 4.1g Carbs: 26.9g

Protein: 20.7g

Salmon and Shrimp Salad

Preparation time: 5 minutes
Cooking time: 0 minutes
Servings: 4

Ingredients:

1 cup smoked salmon, boneless and flaked

1 cup shrimp, peeled, deveined and cooked

½ cup baby arugula

1 tablespoon lemon juice

2 spring onions, chopped

1 tablespoon olive oil

A pinch of sea salt and black pepper

Directions:

In a salad bowl, combine the salmon with the shrimp and the other ingredients, toss and serve.

Nutrition:

Calories: 210

Fat: 6g

Fiber: 5g

Carbs: 10g

Protein: 12g

Shrimp, Tomato and Dates Salad

Preparation time: 10 minutes
Cooking time: 0 minutes
Servings: 4

Ingredients:

1 pound shrimp, cooked, peeled and deveined

2 cups baby spinach

2 tablespoons walnuts, chopped

1 cup cherry tomatoes, halved

1 tablespoon lemon juice

½ cup dates, chopped

2 tablespoons avocado oil

Directions:

In a salad bowl, mix the shrimp with the spinach, walnuts and the other ingredients, toss and serve.

Nutrition:

Calories: 243

Fat: 5.4g

Fiber: 3.3g

Carbs: 21.6g

Protein: 28.3g

Salmon and Watercress Salad

Preparation time: 10 minutes
Cooking time: 0 minutes
Servings: 4

Ingredients:

1 pound smoked salmon, boneless, skinless and flaked

2 spring onions, chopped

2 tablespoons avocado oil

½ cup baby arugula

1 cup watercress

1 tablespoon lemon juice

1 cucumber, sliced

1 avocado, peeled, pitted and roughly cubed

A pinch of sea salt and black pepper

Directions:

In a salad bowl, mix the salmon with the spring onions, watercress and the other ingredients, toss and serve.

Nutrition:

Calories: 261

Fat: 15.8g

Fiber: 4.4g

Carbs: 8.2g

Protein: 22.7g

Apples and Cabbage Mix

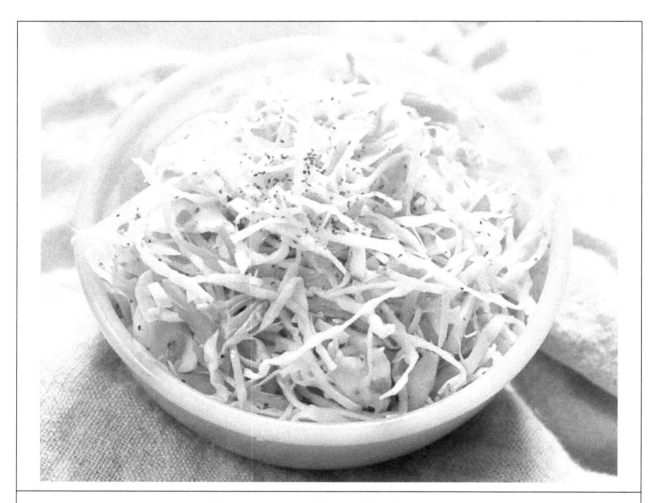

Preparation time: 5 minutes
Cooking time: 0 minutes
Servings: 4

Ingredients:

2 cored and cubed green apples

2 tablespoons Balsamic vinegar

½ tablespoon. Caraway seeds

2 tablespoons olive oil

Black pepper

1 shredded red cabbage head

Directions:

In a bowl, combine the cabbage with the apples and the other ingredients, toss and serve.

Nutrition:

Calories: 165

Fat: 7.4g

Carbs: 26g

Protein: 2.6g

Sugars: 2.6g

Sodium: 19mg

Thyme Mushrooms

Preparation time: 10 minutes
Cooking time: 30 minute
Servings: 4

Ingredients:

1 tablespoon chopped thyme

2 tablespoon olive oil

2 tablespoons chopped parsley

4 minced garlic cloves

Black pepper

2 lbs. halved white mushrooms

Directions:

In a baking pan, combine the mushrooms with the garlic and the other ingredients, toss, introduce in the oven and cook at 400 0F for 30 minutes.

Divide between plates and serve.

Nutrition:

Calories: 251

Fat: 9.3g

Carbs: 13.2 g

Protein: 6 g

Sugars: 0.8 g

Sodium: 37 mg

Rosemary Endives

Preparation time: 5 minutes
Cooking time: 20 minutes
Servings: 4

Ingredients:

2 tablespoons olive oil

1tablespoon dried rosemary

2 halved endives

¼ tablespoon black pepper

½ tablespoon turmeric powder

Directions:

In a baking pan, combine the endives with the oil and the other ingredients, toss gently, introduce in the oven and bake at 400 0F for 20 minutes.

Divide between plates and serve.

Nutrition:

Calories: 66

Fat: 7.1g

Carbs: 1.2 g

Protein: 0.3g

Sugars: 1.3g

Sodium: 113mg

Roasted Beets

Preparation time: 10 minutes
Cooking time: 30 minutes
Servings: 4

Ingredients:

2 minced garlic cloves

¼ teaspoon. Black pepper

4 peeled and sliced beets

¼ c. chopped walnuts

2 tablespoons olive oil

¼ c. chopped parsley

Directions:

In a baking dish, combine the beets with the oil and the other ingredients, toss to coat, introduce in the oven at 420 0F, and bake for 30 minutes.

Divide between plates and serve.

Nutrition:

Calories: 156

Fat: 11.8g

Carbs: 11.5g

Protein: 3.8g

Sugars: 8g,

Sodium: 670 mg

Minty Tomatoes and Corn

Preparation time: 5 minutes
Cooking time: 0 minutes
Servings: 4

Ingredients:

2 c. corn

1 tablespoon rosemary vinegar

2 tablespoons chopped mint

1 lb. sliced tomatoes

¼ tablespoon black pepper

2 tablespoons olive oil

Directions:

In a salad bowl, combine the tomatoes with the corn and the other ingredients, toss and serve.

Enjoy!

Nutrition:

Calories: 230

Fat: 7.2g

Carbs: 11.6g

Protein: 4g

Sugars: 1g

Sodium: 53 mg

Chapter 3 Dinner Recipes

Chicken and Arugula Salad with Italian Dressing

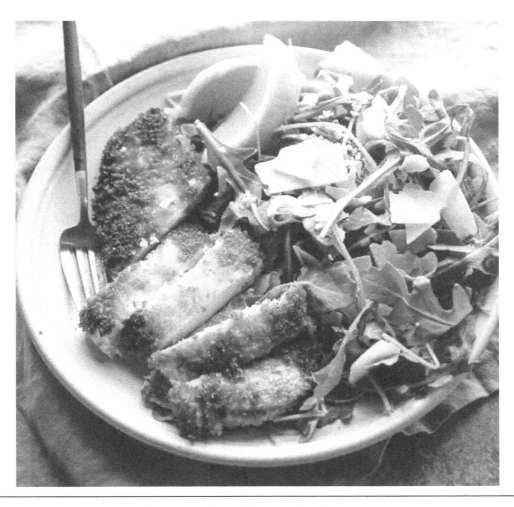

Preparation time: 5 minutes
Cooking time: 30 minutes
Servings: 3

Ingredients:

6oz. of chicken (or turkey), skinless, boneless grilled or prepared in the skillet

Large mixed arugula and lettuce salad

½ cup Italian dressing

½ teaspoon of mustard

Tuna with arugula salad with Italian dressing

6 oz. Can of tuna, drained.

Large mixed arugula

Red onion salad

½ cup Italian dressing

½ teaspoon of mustard

You may use fish sauce instead of salt

Directions:

Mix all the ingredients in a bowl

Nutrition:

Calories: 124 Net carbs: 4.4g Fat: 2.6g

Avocado and Chicken Risotto

Preparation time: 5 minutes
Cooking time: 20 minutes
Servings: 3

Ingredients:

3 cups chicken broth

2 chicken breasts, diced

1 cup risotto rice

2 avocados, peeled and diced

3 teaspoons extra virgin olive oil

1 onion, finely chopped

2 garlic cloves, crushed

2 tablespoons raisins

1 cup grated parmesan cheese, plus extra to serve

5-6 green onions, finely cut, to serve

Directions:

Place chicken broth in a saucepan, bring to the boil, then reduce heat to low and keep at a simmer.

In a non-stick fry pan, cook chicken for 5-6 minutes each side, or until browned and cooked through.

Transfer to a plate in the same pan, heat olive oil over medium heat.

Add the onion and cook, stirring, for 1-2 minutes until softened.

Stir in the garlic, then add the rice and cook, stirring, for 1 minute to coat the grains.

Add the broth, a spoonful at a time, stirring occasionally, allowing each spoonful to be absorbed before adding the next.

Simmer until all liquid has absorbed and rice is tender.

Stir in the chicken, parmesan cheese and raisins, then cover and remove from the heat.

Serve in bowls topped with diced avocados, extra parmesan cheese and chopped green onions.

Nutrition:

Calories: 429

Net carbs: 46.8g

Fat: 15.5g

Protein: 23.4g

Chickpea Fritters

Preparation time: 5 minutes
Cooking time: 30 minutes
Servings: 3

Ingredients:

1 can chickpeas, drained

2 chicken breasts, cooked and shredded

2 egg whites

½ cup fresh parsley leaves, very finely cut

1 teaspoon ginger

½ teaspoon black pepper salt, to taste

2 tablespoons coconut oil, for frying

Directions:

Blend the chickpeas in a food processor and combine them with the chicken, egg whites, parsley, and ginger into a smooth batter.

Heat the oil in a frying pan over medium heat.

Using a large shaper, form the batter into fritters.

Cook each one for 2-3 minutes each side or until golden and cooked through.

Nutrition:

Calories: 207

Net carbs: 35.6g

Fat: 3.1g

Fiber: 9.1g

Protein: 10.3g

Brussels Sprouts Egg Skillet

Preparation time: 5 minutes
Cooking time: 30 minutes
Servings: 3

Ingredients:

½lb Brussels sprouts, halved

1 small onion, chopped

10 cherry tomatoes, halved

4 eggs

1 teaspoon extra virgin olive oil

Directions:

In an 8 inch cast iron skillet, heat olive oil over medium heat.

Add in onion and sauté for 1-2 minutes.

Add in Brussels sprouts and tomatoes and season with salt and pepper to taste.

Cook for 3-4 minutes then crack the eggs, cover and cook until egg whites have set, and egg yolk is desired consistency.

Nutrition:

Calories: 194

Net carbs: 18.2g

Fat: 11.4g

Fiber: 3.4g

Protein: 7.1g

Salmon Kebabs

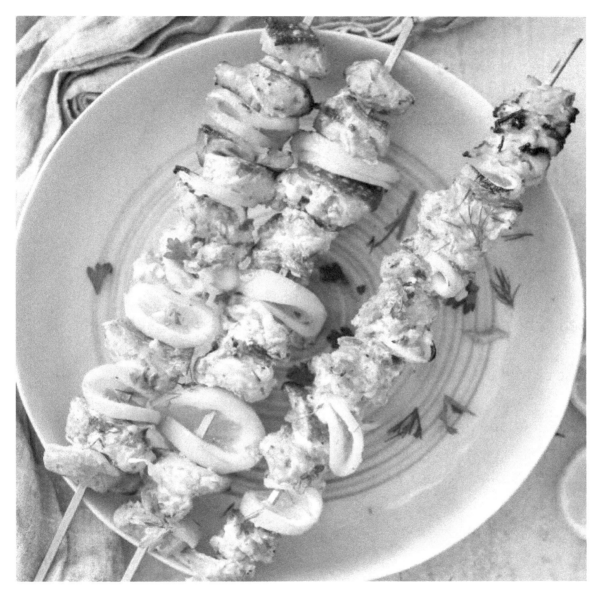

Preparation time: 5 minutes

Cooking time: 20 minutes

Servings: 3

Ingredients:

2 shallots, ends trimmed, halved

2 zucchinis, cut in 2-inch cubes

1 cup cherry tomatoes

6 skinless salmon fillets, cut into 1-inch pieces

3 limes, cut into thin wedges

Directions:

Preheat barbecue or char grill on medium-high.

Thread fish cubes onto skewers, then zucchinis, shallots and tomatoes.

Repeat to make 12 kebabs.

Bake the kebabs for about 3 minutes each side for medium cooked.

Transfer to a plate, cover with foil and set aside for 5 min to rest.

Nutrition:

Calories: 133 Fat: 3.9g Protein: 22.9g

Mediterranean Baked Salmon

Preparation time: 5 minutes
Cooking time: 30 minutes
Servings: 3

Ingredients:

2 (6 Oz) boneless salmon fillets

1 tomato, thinly sliced 1 onion, thinly sliced

1 teaspoon capers 3 teaspoons olive oil

1 teaspoon dry oregano

3g parmesan cheese

Salt and black pepper, to taste

Directions:

Preheat oven to 350F. Place the salmon fillets in a baking dish, sprinkle with oregano, top with onion and tomato slices, drizzle with olive oil, and sprinkle with capers and parmesan cheese. Cover the dish with foil and bake for 30 minutes, or until the fish flakes easily.

Nutrition:

Calories: 197 Protein: 33.3g

Lentil, Kale, and Red Onion Pasta

Preparation time: 10 minutes
Cooking time: 35 minutes
Servings: 2

Ingredients:

2 ½ cups vegetable broth

¾ cup dry lentils

1 bay leaf

¼ cup olive oil

1 large red onion, chopped

1 teaspoon fresh thyme, chopped

½ teaspoon fresh oregano, chopped

8 ounces ground turkey, cut into ¼" slices (optional)

1 bunch kale, stems removed and leaves coarsely chopped

1 (12 ounce) package buckwheat pasta

2 s nutritional yeast

Salt and pepper to taste

Directions:

Rinse the lentils in a fine mesh sieve under cold water until the water runs clear - this will prevent your lentils from getting gummy.

Bring the vegetable broth, lentils, ½ teaspoon of salt, and bay leaf to a boil in a saucepan over high heat. Reduce heat to medium-low, cover, and cook until the lentils are tender, about 20 minutes. Add additional broth if needed to keep the lentils moist. Discard the bay leaf once done.

As the lentils simmer, heat the olive oil in a skillet over medium-high heat. Stir in the onion, thyme, oregano, and season with salt and pepper to taste.

Cook for 1 minute, stirring often, then add the ground turkey, if using. Reduce the heat to medium-low, and cook until the onion has softened, about 10 minutes.

Meanwhile, bring a large pot of lightly salted water to a boil over high heat. Add the kale and pasta. Cook until the pasta is al dente, about 8 minutes.

Remove some of the cooking water and set aside. Drain the pasta, then return to the pot.

Stir in the lentils, and onion mixture.

Use the reserved cooking liquid to adjust the sauciness of the dish to your liking. Sprinkle with nutritional yeast to serve

Nutrition:

Calories: 403 Net carbs: 29.4g Fat: 20.6g

Fiber: 2.1g Protein: 24.6g

Arugula Linguine

Preparation time: 10 minutes
Cooking time: 25 minutes
Servings: 2

Ingredients:

12 ounces linguine or other dried pasta

3 s extra virgin olive oil

3 - 4 cloves garlic, sliced thinly

2 large handfuls baby arugula

2 s capers, drained

½ cup Parmesan, shredded or shaved

1/3 cup pine nuts, toasted

Directions:

Cook the pasta in a large pot of boiling salted water until al dente, about 8 minutes.

While pasta is cooking, heat oil in a large pan and sauté the garlic over medium heat for 2 – 3 minutes until just turning golden.

When your pasta is ready, drain and immediately add the remaining ingredients, including the garlic and toss to combine well.

Nutrition:

Calories: 2

Net carbs: 0.3g

Fiber: 0.2g

Protein: 0.2g

Harvest Nut Roast

Preparation time: 10 minutes
Cooking time: 1 – 1 ½ hours
Servings: 4

Ingredients:

½ cup celery, chopped

2 red onions, chopped ¾ cup walnuts

¾ cup pecan or sunflower meal

2 ½ cups soy milk 1 teaspoon dried basil

1 teaspoon dried lavage

3 cups breadcrumbs

Salt and pepper to taste

Directions:

Preheat oven to 350 degrees F and lightly oil a loaf pan.

In a medium size skillet, sauté the chopped celery and onion in 3 teaspoons water until cooked.

In a large mixing bowl combine the celery and onion with walnuts, pecan or sunflower meal, soy milk, basil, lavage, breadcrumbs, and salt and pepper to taste; mix well.

Place mixture in the prepared loaf pan.

Bake for 60 to 90 minutes; until the loaf is cooked through.

Nutrition:

Calories: 217 Net carbs: 7.7g Fat: 34.3g

Fiber: 0.9g Protein: 3.3g

Shepherd's Pie [Vegan]

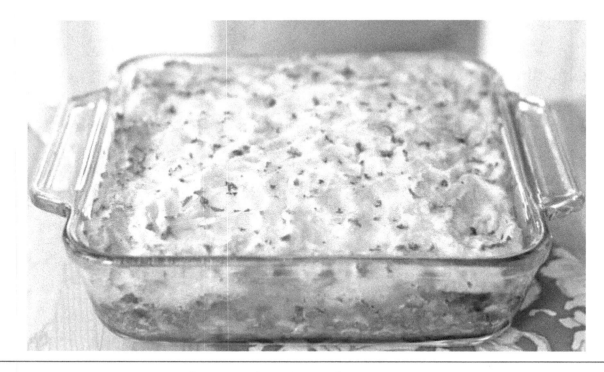

Preparation time: 25 minutes
Cooking time: 1 hour 10 – 20 minutes
Servings: 4

Ingredients:

For the mashed potatoes:

6 large potatoes, peeled and cubed

½ cup soy milk ¼ cup extra virgin olive oil

2 teaspoons salt

For the bottom layer:

1 teaspoon extra virgin olive oil

1 yellow onion, chopped 3 carrots, chopped

3 stalks celery, chopped ½ cup frozen peas

1 tomato, chopped 1 teaspoon dried parsley

1 teaspoon dried lovage

1 teaspoon dried oregano

3 cloves garlic, minced 2/3 cup bulgur

1/2 cup kasha (toasted buckwheat groats)

2 cups fresh mushrooms, diced

Directions:

Preheat oven to 350 degrees F and spray a 2-quart baking dish with cooking spray. Place the potatoes into a large pot with enough cold water to cover them completely. Bring the water to a boil and then reduce heat to a low boil until the potatoes until tender, about 20 minutes. Drain and transfer to a large bowl. Using a hand blender, mix the soy milk, olive oil, and salt into the potatoes, and blend until smooth. Cover and set aside until your bottom layer is ready. At the same time, in a saucepan, bring 1 ½ cups water with ½ teaspoon salt to a boil. Stir in kasha. Reduce heat and simmer uncovered, for 15 minutes. Add 1 ½ cups more water and bring back to a boil. Add bulgur, cover, and remove from heat. Let stand for 10 minutes. Warm the olive oil in a large pan, and sauté the onion, carrots, celery, frozen peas, and tomato on medium heat until they start to soften, about 5 minutes. Add mushrooms and cook for another 3 – 4 minutes. Sprinkle flour over vegetables; stir constantly for 2 minutes or until flour starts to brown. Pour remaining 1 ½ cups milk over the vegetables and increase heat to high. Stir until sauce is smooth. Reduce heat and simmer for 5 minutes. Stir in parsley, lovage, oregano, garlic, and salt and pepper to taste. Combine vegetable mixture and kasha mixture in a large bowl and mix well. Spoon into a greased 10" pie pan, and smooth with a spatula. Spread mashed potatoes over top, leaving an uneven surface. Bake until the potatoes turn golden and the Shepherd's Pie is hot throughout, about 30 minutes

Nutrition:

Calories: 436 Net carbs: 59.6g Fat: 11.4g

Protein: 20.2g

Thai Curry with Chicken and Peanuts

Preparation time: 20 minutes
Cooking time: 20 – 30 minutes
Servings: 4

Ingredients:

2 Bird's Eye chili peppers

2 s ginger root, chopped

1 fresh turmeric root, chopped

½ teaspoon cumin

½ teaspoon dried coriander

1/2 teaspoon ground nutmeg

2 s lemongrass, thinly sliced

1 shallot, chopped

2 cloves garlic, chopped

2 teaspoons fermented shrimp paste

2 s fish sauce

3 s brown sugar

2/3 pound skinless, boneless chicken breast, cut into cubes

2 s extra virgin olive oil

½ cup roasted peanuts

Directions:

Place the chili peppers in a bowl; pour enough water over the chili peppers to cover. Allow the peppers to soak until softened, about 10 minutes. Drain, chop the peppers finely and set aside.

In a large bowl, add the ginger and turmeric root, cumin, coriander, lemongrass, shallot, garlic, shrimp paste, and chopped chili peppers and mash into a paste. Stir the fish sauce and sugar into the paste.

Add the chicken to the paste and toss to coat the evenly.

Cover bowl and marinate for at least 20 minutes, or up to 24 hours in the refrigerator.

Heat the oil in a large skillet over medium heat and cook the chicken until no longer pink in the center and the juices run clear, 5 to 7 minutes.

Stir 2 cups of water into the pan and add the peanuts.

Bring to a simmer and cook until thickened, 20 to 30 minutes. You can also cook this at a lower temperature for up to 2 hours.

Nutrition:

Calories: 426

Net carbs: 52g

Fat: 7.7g

Fiber: 3.9g

Protein: 35g

Red Lentil Curry

Preparation time: 10 minutes
Cooking time: 20 minutes
Servings: 4

Ingredients:

2 cups whole red lentils

1 large red onion, diced

1teaspoon extra virgin olive oil

1 ½ s curry paste

2 s curry powder

1 teaspoon chili powder

1 teaspoon ground turmeric

1 teaspoon ground cumin

1 teaspoon salt

1 teaspoon sugar

3 cloves garlic, minced

1" section of fresh ginger root, peeled and minced

1 (14.25 ounce) can crushed tomatoes

Directions:

Rinse the lentils in a fine mesh sieve under cold water until the water runs clear - this will prevent your lentils from getting gummy.

Transfer the lentils to a medium-sized pot with enough water to cover completely and simmer covered until they're just starting to become tender, about 15 – 20 minutes. Add additional water as necessary.

In the meantime, warm the oil in a large skillet and sauté the onions until they're golden.

In a separate bowl, combine the curry paste, curry powder, chili powder, turmeric, cumin, salt, sugar, garlic, and ginger and mix well.

When the onions are translucent, add the curry mixture and cook on high, stirring constantly for 2 - 3 minutes.

Add in the crushed tomato and reduce the heat. Let the curry blend simmer until the lentils are ready.

When the lentils are cooked to your liking, drain well and add to the curry sauce, mixing well.

Nutrition:

Calories: 323

Net carbs: 36.7g

Fat: 13.2g

Fiber: 14.5g

Protein: 16.4g

Spiced Fish Tacos with Fresh Corn Salsa

Preparation time: 10 minutes
Cooking time: 20 minutes
Servings: 4

Ingredients:

1 cup corn 1/2 cup red onion, diced

1 cup jicama, peeled and chopped

1/2 cup red bell pepper, diced

1 cup fresh cilantro leaves, finely chopped

1 lime, zested and juiced

2 teaspoons sour cream

2 teaspoons cayenne pepper

Salt and pepper to taste 8 fillets tilapia

2 teaspoons olive oil

8 tortillas, warmed

Directions:

Preheat grill for high heat.

For the Corn Salsa: In a medium bowl, mix together corn, red onion, jicama, red bell pepper, and cilantro. Stir in lime juice and zest. Brush each fillet with olive oil, and sprinkle with the cayenne and season to taste. Arrange fillets on grill and cook for 3 minutes per side. For each fish taco, top two corn tortillas with fish, sour cream, and corn salsa.

Nutrition:

Calories: 98 Net carbs: 9.7g Fat: 3.4g

Fiber: 1.4g Protein: 7.4g

Greek Pizza with Arugula, Feta and Olives

Preparation time: 15 minutes
Cooking time: 15 minutes
Servings: 4

Ingredients:

2 tablespoons extra virgin olive oil

4 cloves garlic, minced

3 tablespoons all Purpose flour

1 cup milk

1 teaspoon dried oregano

½ cup Parmesan, grated or shredded

1 cup feta cheese, crumbled

1 (12 inch) pre-baked pizza crust

½ cup oil-packed sun-dried tomatoes, coarsely chopped

2 cups arugula

¼ cup pitted Kalamata olives, coarsely chopped

1/2 small red onion, halved and thinly sliced

1 teaspoon oil from the sun-dried tomatoes

¼ teaspoon chili pepper flakes

Directions:

Adjust oven rack to lowest position, and heat oven to 450 degrees.

For the white sauce: Heat oil in a saucepan and sauté the garlic until it's fragrant, about 2 minutes.

Add the flour and stir well until it's browned, another 2 – 3 minutes.

Add the milk, oregano, Parmesan, and half the Feta and stir continuously until the cheese is well combined and the sauce has thickened, about 5 minutes. Transfer to a small dish.

Assemble the Pizza: Place pizza crust on a cookie sheet; spread white sauce evenly and generously over the crust.

Top with arugula, tomatoes, onions and olives, in that order. Bake until heated through and crisp, about 10 minutes.

Remove from oven, and top with the remaining feta cheese and drizzle oil from the sun-dried tomatoes over top.

Return to oven and bake until cheese melts, about 2 minutes longer. Cut into 8 slices and serve

Nutrition:

Calories: 348

Net carbs: 6.9g Fat: 27.5g

Fiber: 2.6g Protein: 19.6g

Chapter 4 Snacks

Pear, Cranberry And Chocolate Crisp

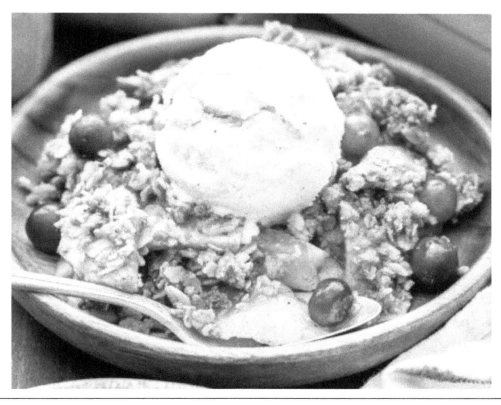

Preparation time: 15 minutes
Cooking time: 40 minutes
Servings: 4

Ingredients:

Crumble topping:

1/2 cup flour

1/2 cup brown sugar

1 teaspoon cinnamon

⅛ Teaspoon salt

3/4 cup yogurt

1/4 cup sliced peppers

1/3 cup butter, melted

1 teaspoon vanilla

Filling:

1 brown sugar

3 teaspoon, cut into balls

1/4 cup dried cranberries

1 teaspoon lemon juice

Two handfuls of milk chocolate chips

Directions:

Preheat oven to 375.

Spray a casserole dish with a butter spray.

Put all of the topping ingredients - flour, sugar, cinnamon, salt, nuts, legumes and dried

Butter a bowl and then mix. Set aside.

In a large bowl combine the sugar, lemon juice, pears, and cranberries.

Once the fully blended move to the prepared baking dish.

Spread the topping evenly over the fruit.

Bake for about half an hour.

Disperse chocolate chips out at the top.

Cook for another 10 minutes.

Have with ice cream.

Nutrition:

Calories: 418 Net carbs: 107.7g

Fat: 0.4g Fiber: 2.8g Protein: 0.5g

Raw Vegan Double Almond Raw Chocolate Tart

Preparation time: 10 minutes
Cooking time: 35 minutes
Servings: 4

Ingredients:

1½ cups of raw almonds

¼ cup of coconut oil, melted

1 raw honey or royal jelly

8 ounces dark chocolate, chopped

1 cup of coconut milk

½ cup unsweetened shredded coconut

Directions:

Crust:

Ground almonds and add melted coconut oil, raw honey and combine.

Using a spatula, spread this mixture into the tart or pie pan.

Filling:

Put the chopped chocolate in a bowl, heat coconut milk and pour over chocolate and whisk together.

Pour filling into tart shell.

Refrigerate.

Toast almond slivers chips and sprinkle over tart.

Nutrition:

Calories: 101 Net carbs: 3.4g Fat: 9.4g

Fiber: 0.6g Protein: 2.4g

Raw Vegan Bounty Bars

Preparation time: 10 minutes
Cooking time: 35 minutes
Servings: 4

Ingredients:

"Peanut" butter filling

2 cups desiccated coconut

3 coconut oil - melted

1 cup of coconut cream - full fat

4 of raw honey

1 teaspoon ground vanilla bean

Pinch of sea salt

Super foods chocolate part:

½ cup cacao powder 2 raw honey

1/3 cup of coconut oil (melted)

Directions:

Mix coconut oil, coconut cream, and honey, vanilla and salt.

Pour over desiccated coconut and mix well.

Mold coconut mixture into balls, small bars similar to bounty and freeze.

Or pour the whole mixture into a tray, freeze and cut into small bars.

Make super foods chocolate mixture, warm it up and dip frozen coconut into the chocolate and put on a tray and freeze again.

Nutrition:

Calories: 70 Net carbs: 6.7g Fat: 4.3g

Fiber: 0.2g Protein: 1g

Raw Vegan Tartlets with Coconut Cream

Preparation time: 10 minutes
Cooking time: 35 minutes
Servings: 4

Ingredients:

Pudding:

1 avocado

2 coconut oil

2 raw honey

2 cacao powder

1 teaspoon ground vanilla bean

Pinch of salt

¼ cup almond milk, as needed

Directions:

Blend all the ingredients in the food processor until smooth and thick.

Spread evenly into tartlet crusts.

Optionally, put some goji berries on top of the pudding layer.

Make the coconut cream, spread it on top of the pudding layer, and put back in the fridge overnight.

Serve with one blueberry on top of each tartlet.

Nutrition:

Calories: 200 Net carbs: 25.2g Fat: 4.3g

Fiber: 4.6g Protein: 12.8g

Raw Vegan "Peanut" Butter Truffles

Preparation time: 10 minutes
Cooking time: 30 minutes
Servings: 4

Ingredients:

5 sunflower seed butter

1 coconut oil

1 raw honey

1 teaspoon ground vanilla bean

¾ cup almond flour

1 flaxseed meal

Pinch of salt

1 cacao butter

Hemp hearts (optional)

¼ cup super-foods chocolate

Directions:

Mix until all ingredients are incorporated.

Roll the dough into 1-inch balls, place them on parchment paper and refrigerate for half an hour (yield about 14 truffles).

Dip each truffle in the melted super foods chocolate, one at the time.

Place them back on the pan with parchment paper or coat them in cocoa powder or coconut flakes.

Nutrition:

Calories: 94 Net carbs: 3.1g Fat: 8g

Fiber: 1g Protein: 4g

Raw Vegan Chocolate Pie

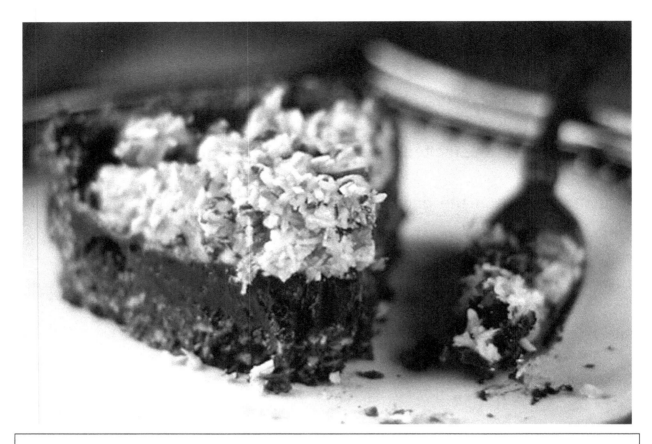

Preparation time: 10 minutes
Cooking time: 25 minutes
Servings: 4

Ingredients: Crust:

2 cups almonds, soaked overnight and drained

1 cup pitted dates, soaked overnight and drained

1 cup chopped dried apricots

1½ teaspoon ground vanilla bean

2 teaspoon chia seeds 1 banana

Filling:

4 raw cacao powder 3 raw honey

2 ripe avocados 2 organic coconut oil

2 almond milk (if needed, check for consistency first)

Directions:

Add almonds and banana to a food processor or blender.

Mix until it forms a thick ball.

Add the vanilla, dates, and apricot chunks to the blender.

Mix well and optionally add a couple of drops of water at a time to make the mixture stick together.

Spread in a 10-inch dis.

Mix filling ingredients in a blender and add almond milk if necessary.

Add filling to the crust and refrigerate.

Nutrition:

Calories: 380

Net carbs: 50.2g

Fat: 18.4g

Fiber: 2.2g

Protein: 7.2g

Apricot Oatmeal Cookies

Preparation time: 10 minutes
Cooking time: 40 minutes
Servings: 7

Ingredients:

1/2 cup (1 stick) butter, softened

2/3 cup light brown sugar packed 1 egg

3/4 cup all-purpose flour

1/2 teaspoon baking soda

1/2 teaspoon vanilla extract

1/2 teaspoon cinnamon 1/4 teaspoon salt

1 teaspoon 1/2 cups chopped oats

3/4 cup yolks 1/4 cup sliced apricots

1/3 cup slivered almonds

Directions:

Preheat oven to 350°. In a big bowl combine with the butter, sugar, and egg until smooth. In another bowl whisk the flour, baking soda, cinnamon, and salt together. Stir the dry ingredients to the butter-sugar bowl. Now stir in the oats, raisins, apricots, and almonds.

I heard on the web that in this time, it's much better to cool with the dough (therefore, your biscuits are thicker)

Nutrition:

Calories: 196 Net carbs: 30g

Fat: 8.1g Fiber: 0.5g Protein: 3g

Raw Vegan Reese's Cups

Preparation time: 10 minutes
Cooking time: 35 minutes
Servings: 4

Ingredients:

"Peanut" butter filling

½ cup sunflower seeds butter

½ cup almond butter

1 raw honey

2 melted coconut oil

Super foods chocolate part:

½ cup cacao powder

2 raw honey

1/3 cup of coconut oil (melted)

Directions:

Mix the "peanut" butter filling ingredients.

Put a spoonful of the mixture into each muffin cup.

Refrigerate.

Mix super foods chocolate ingredients.

Put a spoonful of the super foods chocolate mixture over the "peanut" butter mixture. Freeze!

Nutrition:

Calories: 549 Net carbs: 54g Fat: 31.7g

Fiber: 2.1g Protein: 11.8g

Raw Vegan Coffee Cashew Cream Cake

Preparation time: 10 minutes
Cooking time: 35 minutes
Servings: 4

Ingredients:

Coffee cashew cream

2 cups raw cashews

1 teaspoon of ground vanilla bean

3 melted coconut oil

¼ cup raw honey

1/3 cup very strong coffee or triple espresso shot

Directions:

Blend all ingredients for the cream, pour it onto the crust and refrigerate.

Garnish with coffee beans.

Nutrition:

Calories: 94

Net carbs: 4.4g

Fat: 7.9g

Fiber: 0.3g

Protein: 2.8g

Raw Vegan Chocolate Cashew Truffles

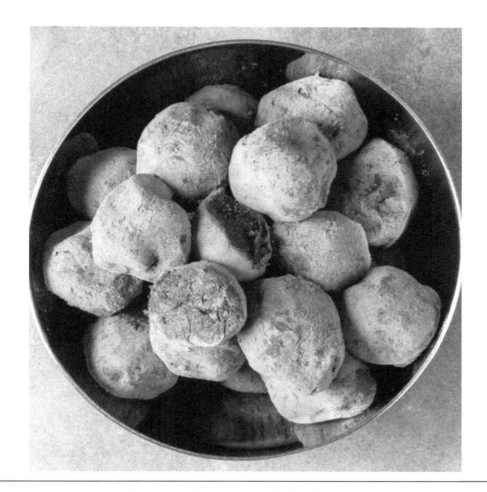

Preparation time: 10 minutes
Cooking time: 35 minutes
Servings: 4

Ingredients:

1 cup ground cashews

1 teaspoon of ground vanilla bean

½ cup of coconut oil

¼ cup raw honey

2 flax meal

2 hemp hearts

2 cacao powder

Directions:

Mix all ingredients and make truffles. Sprinkle coconut flakes on top.

Nutrition:

Calories: 87

Net carbs: 6g

Fat: 6.5g

Fiber: 0.5g

Protein: 2.3g

Raw Vegan Chocolate Walnut Truffles

Preparation time: 10 minutes
Cooking time: 35 minutes
Servings: 4

Ingredients:

1 cup ground walnuts

1 teaspoon cinnamon

½ cup of coconut oil

¼ cup raw honey

2 chia seeds

2 cacao powder

Directions:

Mix all ingredients and make truffles.

Coat with cinnamon, coconut flakes or chopped almonds.

Nutrition:

Calories: 120

Fat: 13.6g

Fat: 0.2g

Fiber: 0.5g

Protein: 7g

Conclusion

I wish you appreciated my yummy dishes.

Thanks for checking out guide as well as reaching this factor.

Bear in mind that for ideal outcomes, dishes must be attempted a couple of times to tweak the dish to your home appliances.

Keep risk-free as well as knowingly consume healthy and balanced and also healthy foods, your body is your holy place, treat it the very best you can.

For a full dish strategy get in touch with a physician and also live life with happiness.

See you quickly with this remarkable diet regimen.

CPSIA information can be obtained
at www.ICGtesting.com
Printed in the USA
LVHW062338230421
685368LV00004B/308

9 781667 159720